Flourishing Without Gluten: A Comprehensive Guide to Gluten-Free Living

Chapter 1: Understanding Gluten and Celiac Disease
- Introduction to gluten and its role in food
- Explanation of celiac disease and gluten intolerance
- Symptoms and effects of celiac disease on the body
- Diagnosis and testing for celiac disease

Chapter 2: The Basics of Gluten-Free Living
- Transitioning to a gluten-free diet
- Identifying gluten-containing foods
- Reading food labels for hidden gluten

- Hope for a future with greater understanding and acceptance of gluten intolerance

Conclusion: Embracing Your Gluten-Free Journey
- Reflecting on the journey to gluten-free living
- Celebrating the victories and milestones along the way
- Encouragement for continued growth and adaptation in the gluten-free lifestyle
- A reminder that living gluten-free can be empowering and fulfilling

Prologue: A Gluten-Free Love Story

In the hustle and bustle of life's unpredictable journey, fate often presents us with unexpected twists and turns. For me, a young professional navigating the complexities of career and personal life, one such twist came in the form of a chance encounter that would change the course of my life forever.

It was a crisp autumn day when I first laid eyes on Laura, a vibrant and captivating woman with a smile that could light up the darkest of rooms. Our meeting was serendipitous, a collision of worlds that seemed predestined by the hand of fate. Little did I know that this chance encounter would not only lead to a deep and enduring love but also introduce me to the world of gluten intolerance in a way I never imagined.

As our relationship blossomed and grew, I soon discovered that Laura had been living with gluten intolerance for most of her life. From dining out at restaurants to grocery shopping and meal planning, gluten-free living had become second nature to her. Intrigued by Laura's resilience and determination, I delved into the world of gluten-free living, eager to learn more about her dietary needs and how I could support her on this journey.

Our love story unfolded against the backdrop of gluten-free dinners, shared recipes, and moments of laughter and understanding. As we dreamed of building a future together, I couldn't shake the lingering thought that our potential children might inherit Laura's gluten intolerance. It was a concern that weighed heavily on my mind, sparking conversations about the challenges and uncertainties we might face as a family.

Despite the unknowns that lay ahead, Laura and my love only grew stronger, fortified by our shared experiences and unwavering commitment to each other. As we embarked on the adventure of parenthood, we faced each challenge with courage and optimism, knowing that together, we could overcome anything life threw our way.

And so begins the story of Laura and I—a love story intertwined with the complexities of gluten intolerance, resilience, and the boundless possibilities of the future. As they journey through life together, we discover that love knows no bounds and that true strength lies in facing life's challenges hand in hand, with hearts full of

hope and a shared determination to
embrace whatever the future may hold.

Chapter 1: Understanding Gluten and Its Role in Food

Gluten is a protein found in certain grains, notably wheat, barley, and rye. It plays a crucial role in the texture, structure, and elasticity of many foods. Understanding the function of gluten in food is essential for those seeking to adopt a gluten-free lifestyle.

1.1 What is Gluten?

Gluten is composed of two main proteins: glutenin and gliadin. When flour is mixed with water, these proteins combine to form a sticky network that gives dough its elastic properties. This elasticity allows bread to rise and gives it a chewy texture.

1.2 Gluten-Containing Grains

The primary sources of gluten in the diet are wheat, barley, and rye. These grains are commonly used in a wide range of foods, including bread, pasta, cereals, baked goods, and processed foods. It's important to carefully read food labels, as gluten can hide in unexpected places, such as sauces, soups, and even some medications.

1.3 Functions of Gluten in Food
Gluten serves several important functions in food production:

- Structure: Gluten provides the framework that allows bread and other baked goods to rise and maintain their shape during baking.
- Texture: Gluten gives baked goods their characteristic chewiness and springiness.
- Binding: Gluten helps ingredients stick together in recipes like meatballs, veggie burgers, and meatloaf.

- Moisture retention: Gluten helps retain moisture in baked goods, preventing them from becoming dry and crumbly.

1.4 Gluten in Food Processing
Gluten is often added to processed foods as a thickening agent, stabilizer, or flavor enhancer. It can also be used as a coating for fried foods to create a crispy texture. In addition, gluten-derived ingredients such as wheat starch, malt extract, and hydrolyzed wheat protein are commonly used in food manufacturing.

1.5 Health Implications of Gluten
While gluten is harmless for most people, it can cause adverse reactions in individuals with celiac disease, wheat allergy, or non-celiac gluten sensitivity. Celiac disease is an autoimmune disorder triggered by the ingestion of gluten, resulting in damage to the small intestine and various symptoms

such as digestive issues, fatigue, and skin problems. Wheat allergy is an immune response to proteins found in wheat, including gluten, which can cause symptoms ranging from hives and itching to life-threatening anaphylaxis. Non-celiac gluten sensitivity is a condition characterized by symptoms similar to those of celiac disease but without the autoimmune component.

1.6 In summary, gluten plays a crucial role in the texture, structure, and functionality of many foods. While it is harmless for most people, those with celiac disease, wheat allergy, or non-celiac gluten sensitivity must avoid gluten-containing grains and products to prevent adverse health effects. Understanding the role of gluten in food is the first step towards adopting a gluten-free lifestyle and making informed dietary choices.

Chapter 2: The Basics of Living Gluten-Free

Living gluten-free involves more than just avoiding certain foods; it requires a fundamental shift in dietary habits and lifestyle choices. In this chapter, we'll explore the essential aspects of gluten-free living, from understanding gluten-containing foods to practical tips for grocery shopping and meal planning.

2.1 Understanding Gluten and Gluten-Free Foods

To live gluten-free successfully, it's crucial to understand what gluten is and which foods contain it. Gluten is a protein found in wheat, barley, rye, and their derivatives. This includes common foods like bread, pasta, cereal, and baked goods. However, gluten can also hide in less obvious places, such as sauces, marinades, and processed meats. Learning to read food labels carefully and familiarizing yourself with gluten-free alternatives is key.

2.2 Transitioning to a Gluten-Free Diet
Transitioning to a gluten-free diet can be challenging, especially for those accustomed to eating gluten-containing foods. It's essential to approach the transition with patience and an open mind. Start by gradually eliminating gluten-containing foods from your diet and replacing them with gluten-free alternatives. Experiment with new recipes and ingredients to discover what works best for you.

2.3 Identifying Gluten-Free Foods
Fortunately, there are plenty of naturally gluten-free foods to enjoy, including fruits, vegetables, lean proteins, dairy products, and gluten-free grains like rice, quinoa, and

corn. Focus on building meals around these wholesome, naturally gluten-free ingredients. Additionally, many manufacturers offer certified gluten-free products, which undergo rigorous testing to ensure they meet gluten-free standards.

2.4 Reading Food Labels

When shopping for gluten-free products, it's essential to become proficient at reading food labels. Look for products labeled "gluten-free" or with a gluten-free certification logo. Be wary of ingredients like wheat, barley, rye, and malt, as well as less obvious sources of gluten such as modified food starch and hydrolyzed vegetable protein. If you're unsure whether a product is gluten-free, contact the manufacturer for clarification.

2.5 Meal Planning and Preparation

Meal planning is a crucial aspect of successful gluten-free living. Take time each week to plan your meals and snacks, making sure to include a variety of gluten-free foods to ensure balanced nutrition. Stock your pantry with gluten-free staples like rice, quinoa, gluten-free pasta, and flour alternatives. Invest in gluten-free cookbooks or explore online resources for inspiration and recipe ideas.

2.6 Dining Out and Social Situations
Eating out can present challenges for those following a gluten-free diet, but with some preparation and communication, it's entirely possible to enjoy dining out safely. Research restaurants ahead of time to find gluten-free options and inform your server about your dietary restrictions. Many restaurants now offer gluten-free menus or are willing to accommodate special requests. When attending social gatherings

or events, consider bringing a gluten-free dish to share to ensure you have safe options available.

2.7 Living gluten-free requires education, preparation, and a willingness to adapt. By understanding the basics of gluten-free living, including identifying gluten-containing foods, reading food labels, and mastering meal planning and preparation, you can navigate the gluten-free lifestyle with confidence and ease. Remember that living gluten-free isn't just about what you can't eat—it's about embracing a healthy, vibrant way of eating that nourishes your body and soul.

Chapter 3: Gluten-Free Cooking Techniques

Cooking gluten-free doesn't have to mean sacrificing flavor or texture. With the right techniques and ingredients, you can create delicious, satisfying meals that everyone will enjoy. In this chapter, we'll explore various gluten-free cooking techniques, from alternative flours and grains to tips for successful gluten-free baking.

3.1 Alternative Flours and Grains

One of the first steps in gluten-free cooking is familiarizing yourself with alternative flours and grains. While wheat flour is off-limits, there are many gluten-free flours and grains that can be used in its place. Some popular options include:

- Rice flour: Made from finely ground rice, rice flour is versatile and has a mild flavor,

making it suitable for both sweet and savory recipes.
- Almond flour: Made from blanched almonds, almond flour adds a rich, nutty flavor and moist texture to baked goods.
- Coconut flour: Made from dried coconut meat, coconut flour is high in fiber and adds a subtle coconut flavor to recipes.
- Quinoa flour: Ground from quinoa seeds, quinoa flour is high in protein and has a nutty flavor, making it ideal for baking.

Experiment with different flours and grains to find the ones you enjoy working with and the ones that best suit your recipes.

3.2 Baking Without Gluten
Baking without gluten requires some adjustments to traditional baking techniques, but with practice, you can achieve delicious results. Here are some tips for successful gluten-free baking:

- Use a blend of gluten-free flours: Mix different gluten-free flours to create a blend that mimics the properties of wheat flour. A common blend includes a combination of rice flour, potato starch, tapioca flour, and xanthan gum.
- Add binders and leavening agents: Since gluten provides structure and elasticity in baked goods, it's essential to add binders like xanthan gum or guar gum to help hold the ingredients together. Additionally, use leavening agents like baking powder or baking soda to help baked goods rise.
- Increase moisture: Gluten-free flours tend to absorb more moisture than wheat flour, so it's often necessary to increase the liquid content in recipes. Add extra eggs, milk, or other liquids to ensure your baked goods stay moist and tender.

3.3 Substituting Ingredients

When adapting recipes to be gluten-free, it's essential to substitute gluten-containing ingredients with suitable alternatives. Here are some common substitutions:

- Wheat flour: Replace wheat flour with gluten-free flours like rice flour, almond flour, or coconut flour. Keep in mind that gluten-free flours have different properties, so you may need to adjust the quantities and proportions in your recipes.
- Bread crumbs: Use gluten-free breadcrumbs made from rice or cornmeal instead of traditional breadcrumbs.
- Soy sauce: Opt for gluten-free tamari or coconut aminos as a soy sauce substitute in recipes.
- Thickening agents: Use cornstarch, arrowroot powder, or tapioca flour as thickening agents in soups, sauces, and gravies instead of wheat flour.

3.4 Creating Balanced and Nutritious Meals
A gluten-free diet can be nutritious and balanced when you focus on incorporating a variety of whole foods into your meals. Fill your plate with plenty of fruits, vegetables, lean proteins, and gluten-free grains like quinoa, brown rice, and buckwheat. Experiment with different cooking techniques, such as grilling, roasting, steaming, and sautéing, to enhance the flavors and textures of your dishes.

3.5 Cooking gluten-free requires creativity, experimentation, and a willingness to try new ingredients and techniques. By familiarizing yourself with alternative flours and grains, mastering the art of gluten-free baking, and substituting ingredients in recipes as needed, you can create delicious, satisfying meals that cater to your dietary needs and preferences. With practice and patience, gluten-free cooking can become second nature, allowing you to enjoy a diverse and flavorful diet without gluten.

Chapter 4: Dining Out and Traveling Gluten-Free

Maintaining a gluten-free diet while dining out or traveling can present unique challenges, but with careful planning and communication, it's entirely possible to enjoy delicious meals and explore new culinary experiences. In this chapter, we'll explore strategies for dining out safely and navigating gluten-free options while traveling.

4.1 Researching Restaurants and Establishments

Before dining out, it's helpful to research restaurants and establishments that offer gluten-free options. Many restaurants now provide gluten-free menus or indicate gluten-free options on their regular menus. Websites and review platforms often include information about restaurants' gluten-free offerings and accommodations, making it easier to find suitable dining options.

4.2 Communicating with Restaurant Staff

When dining out gluten-free, communication with restaurant staff is key. Inform your server about your dietary restrictions and ask questions about menu items and preparation methods. Be specific about your needs, including cross-contamination concerns, and politely request accommodations as needed. Most restaurants are willing to accommodate special dietary requests and can provide guidance on safe options.

4.3 Navigating Menus and Making Substitutions

When perusing menus, look for naturally gluten-free options or dishes that can be easily modified to be gluten-free. Choose simple, whole foods like grilled meats, seafood, vegetables, and salads, and avoid dishes with breaded or fried components. Don't hesitate to ask for substitutions or modifications to accommodate your dietary needs, such as swapping out pasta for gluten-free pasta or requesting a gluten-free bun for burgers or sandwiches.

4.4 Being Mindful of Cross-Contamination
Cross-contamination is a significant concern for those with gluten intolerance or celiac disease, as even small traces of gluten can cause adverse reactions. When dining out, be vigilant about potential sources of cross-contamination, such as shared cooking surfaces, utensils, and fryers. Ask about kitchen practices and protocols for preventing cross-contact with gluten-containing ingredients, and choose restaurants with a reputation for accommodating gluten-free diners safely.

4.5 Packable Snacks and Meals for Travel
When traveling gluten-free, it's essential to pack plenty of snacks and meals to ensure you have safe options available, especially during long flights or road trips. Pack portable snacks like nuts, seeds, dried fruit, gluten-free granola bars, and rice cakes to keep hunger at bay while on the go. Consider bringing pre-made meals or ingredients for assembling quick and easy gluten-free meals, such as salads, sandwiches made with gluten-free bread, and rice or quinoa bowls.

4.6 Researching Local Cuisine and Ingredients
Before traveling to a new destination, take the time to research local cuisine and ingredients to better understand what options may be available to you. Learn about traditional gluten-free dishes and

ingredients commonly used in the region, and familiarize yourself with any language barriers or cultural differences that may impact your dining experience. Consider reaching out to local celiac support groups or online communities for recommendations and tips from fellow gluten-free travelers.

4.7 Conclusion

Dining out and traveling gluten-free requires careful planning, communication, and flexibility, but it's entirely possible to enjoy delicious meals and memorable culinary experiences while adhering to a gluten-free diet. By researching restaurants and establishments, communicating with restaurant staff, making mindful menu choices, and being prepared with packable snacks and meals for travel, you can navigate dining out and traveling with confidence and ease. Remember to prioritize your health and safety while exploring new foods and destinations, and don't hesitate to advocate for your dietary needs when necessary.

Chapter 5: Gluten-Free Management of Social Situations and Special Occasions

Navigating social situations and special occasions while living gluten-free can present unique challenges, but with preparation, communication, and a positive mindset, you can participate fully in gatherings and celebrations without compromising your dietary needs. In this chapter, we'll explore strategies for managing social situations and special occasions while maintaining a gluten-free lifestyle.

5.1 Handling Social Gatherings and Parties
Social gatherings and parties often revolve around food, making them potential minefields for those with gluten intolerance or celiac disease. However, with some planning and foresight, you can navigate

these situations successfully. Here are some tips:

- Communicate with the host: If you're attending a gathering at someone's home, don't hesitate to reach out to the host ahead of time to discuss your dietary needs. Offer to bring a gluten-free dish to share or ask if they can accommodate your needs with gluten-free options.
- Eat before you go: If you're unsure whether there will be safe options available, consider eating a small meal or snack before the event to curb your hunger and minimize the temptation to indulge in potentially unsafe foods.
- Bring your own snacks: Always come prepared with gluten-free snacks or portable foods to ensure you have safe options available. Pack items like nuts, seeds, fruit, or gluten-free granola bars to munch on throughout the event.

5.2 Educating Friends and Family

Educating friends and family about your dietary needs is essential for garnering their support and understanding. Many people may not be familiar with gluten intolerance or celiac disease and may inadvertently offer you foods that contain gluten. Take the time to explain your condition and the importance of avoiding gluten, and provide guidance on safe options they can offer you when hosting gatherings or meals.

5.3 Celebrating Holidays and Special Occasions

Holidays and special occasions can be particularly challenging for those living gluten-free, as traditional foods and customs often revolve around gluten-containing dishes. However, with a bit of creativity and adaptation, you can still enjoy festive celebrations without compromising your dietary needs. Here are some strategies:

- Modify traditional recipes: Adapt your favorite holiday recipes to be gluten-free by substituting gluten-containing ingredients with suitable alternatives. Experiment with gluten-free flours, breadcrumbs, and sauces to recreate the flavors and textures of traditional dishes.
- Host your own gathering: Take control of the menu by hosting your own gluten-free holiday feast or special occasion celebration. Invite friends and family to join you in preparing and enjoying delicious gluten-free dishes together.
- Focus on the spirit of the occasion: Remember that holidays and special occasions are about more than just food— they're opportunities to connect with loved ones, create lasting memories, and celebrate traditions. Focus on the joy and

camaraderie of the event rather than fixating on what you can't eat.

5.4 Coping with Emotional Challenges

Living gluten-free in a gluten-filled world can sometimes evoke feelings of frustration, isolation, or anxiety, especially in social situations or during special occasions. It's essential to acknowledge and address these emotions and find healthy coping mechanisms to navigate them. Seek support from friends, family, or online communities of fellow gluten-free individuals who can offer empathy, understanding, and practical advice. Practice self-care techniques such as mindfulness, meditation, or engaging in activities that bring you joy and relaxation.

5.5 Conclusion

Managing social situations and special occasions while living gluten-free requires planning, communication, and a positive attitude. By advocating for your dietary needs, educating friends and family, adapting recipes to be gluten-free, and focusing on the joy of the occasion rather than the food, you can participate fully in gatherings and celebrations without compromising your health or well-being. Remember that you are not alone in your gluten-free journey, and with support and resilience, you can navigate any social situation or special occasion with confidence and grace.

Chapter 6: Gluten-Free Nutrition and Health

Maintaining a balanced and nutritious diet is essential for overall health and well-being, especially for those living with gluten intolerance or celiac disease. In this chapter, we'll explore the unique nutritional considerations and health implications of a gluten-free lifestyle, as well as strategies for ensuring optimal nutrition while avoiding gluten.

6.1 Ensuring a Balanced Diet

One of the primary concerns for individuals following a gluten-free diet is ensuring they receive adequate nutrition. Gluten-free foods can sometimes be lower in certain nutrients, such as fiber, iron, calcium, and B vitamins, compared to their gluten-containing counterparts. To mitigate this, focus on incorporating a variety of nutrient-dense foods into your diet, including fruits, vegetables, lean proteins, dairy or dairy alternatives, and gluten-free grains like quinoa, brown rice, and buckwheat. Aim for a balanced mix of macronutrients—carbohydrates, protein, and healthy fats—to support your energy levels and overall health.

6.2 Addressing Nutrient Deficiencies
Individuals with celiac disease are at increased risk of nutrient deficiencies due to malabsorption and damage to the small intestine. Common nutrient deficiencies associated with celiac disease include iron, calcium, vitamin D, vitamin B12, folate, and zinc. To address these deficiencies, consider working with a registered dietitian or healthcare provider to develop a personalized nutrition plan that includes appropriate supplementation, fortified

foods, and dietary strategies to optimize nutrient absorption.

6.3 Supplements and Vitamins
Supplements and vitamins can be valuable tools for filling nutritional gaps in a gluten-free diet, especially for individuals with celiac disease or other conditions that affect nutrient absorption. Some common supplements to consider include:

- Iron: Iron deficiency is common in individuals with celiac disease, so iron supplementation may be necessary to correct deficiencies and prevent anemia.
- Calcium and vitamin D: Since dairy products are a significant source of calcium and vitamin D in the diet, those who avoid dairy due to lactose intolerance or other reasons may need to supplement to meet their needs.

- B vitamins: B vitamins, including B12 and folate, are essential for energy metabolism, nerve function, and red blood cell production. Consider supplementing with a B-complex vitamin to ensure adequate intake.
- Probiotics: Probiotics can help support digestive health and alleviate symptoms of gastrointestinal discomfort commonly experienced by individuals with celiac disease or gluten intolerance.

6.4 Impact of Gluten-Free Living on Overall Well-Being
Adopting a gluten-free lifestyle can have both positive and negative effects on overall well-being, depending on individual circumstances and dietary choices. While eliminating gluten-containing foods may alleviate symptoms and improve digestive health for those with celiac disease or gluten intolerance, it's essential to ensure

that gluten-free substitutions are nutritious and balanced. Additionally, the social and emotional aspects of living gluten-free, such as navigating social situations, managing stress, and coping with the psychological impact of dietary restrictions, can impact overall well-being. Practicing self-care techniques, seeking support from healthcare professionals and support groups, and maintaining a positive attitude can help promote emotional and mental well-being while living gluten-free.

6.5 Conclusion
Navigating nutrition and health while living gluten-free requires education, awareness, and proactive management. By focusing on a balanced diet, addressing nutrient deficiencies, considering supplementation when necessary, and prioritizing overall well-being, you can optimize your health and thrive on a gluten-free diet. Remember

that each person's nutritional needs are unique, so it's essential to work with healthcare professionals to develop a personalized nutrition plan tailored to your individual needs and circumstances. With proper guidance and support, you can enjoy a vibrant and fulfilling life while managing gluten intolerance or celiac disease with confidence.

Chapter 7: Gluten-Free for Kids and Families

Raising a child with gluten intolerance or celiac disease requires careful planning, education, and support from the entire family. In this chapter, we'll explore the unique challenges and considerations of living gluten-free as a family, as well as strategies for ensuring a safe and enjoyable gluten-free lifestyle for children.

7.1 Understanding Gluten Intolerance in Children

Gluten intolerance, including celiac disease and non-celiac gluten sensitivity, can present unique challenges for children and their families. Celiac disease is an autoimmune disorder triggered by gluten consumption, resulting in damage to the small intestine and various symptoms, including digestive issues, fatigue, and failure to thrive. Non-celiac gluten sensitivity is a condition characterized by symptoms similar to those of celiac disease but without the autoimmune component. It's essential for parents and caregivers to understand the signs and symptoms of gluten intolerance in children and work closely with healthcare professionals to obtain an accurate diagnosis and develop a management plan.

7.2 Transitioning to a Gluten-Free Diet

Transitioning a child to a gluten-free diet can be challenging, especially if they're accustomed to eating gluten-containing foods. It's essential to approach the transition with sensitivity and empathy, explaining to your child why certain foods need to be avoided and reassuring them that there are plenty of delicious gluten-free alternatives available. Involve your child in meal planning and preparation, allowing them to explore new gluten-free foods and recipes and empowering them to make healthy choices.

7.3 Creating a Gluten-Free Home Environment
Creating a gluten-free home environment is crucial for minimizing the risk of cross-contamination and ensuring a safe and supportive space for your child. Here are some tips for establishing a gluten-free home:

- Remove gluten-containing foods from your pantry and refrigerator to eliminate temptation and reduce the risk of accidental ingestion.
- Use separate utensils, cutting boards, and cooking equipment for gluten-free and gluten-containing foods to prevent cross-contact.

- Label gluten-free foods clearly and store them in designated areas to avoid confusion.
- Educate other family members, caregivers, and visitors about the importance of maintaining a gluten-free environment and the steps necessary to prevent cross-contamination.

7.4 Advocating for Gluten-Free Accommodations

Advocating for gluten-free accommodations in schools, daycare facilities, and social settings is essential for ensuring your child's safety and well-being. Work closely with school administrators, teachers, and food service staff to develop a plan for accommodating your child's dietary needs, including providing gluten-free meal options in the cafeteria, implementing safe food handling practices, and educating staff and students about gluten intolerance. Encourage open communication and collaboration to address any concerns or challenges that may arise.

7.5 Supporting Children Emotionally and Socially

Living with gluten intolerance can impact children emotionally and socially, especially as they navigate social situations and peer relationships. It's essential to provide emotional support and encouragement to help your child cope with the challenges of living gluten-free. Encourage open communication and create opportunities for your child to connect with other children who are also living gluten-free, whether through support groups, online communities, or social events. Foster a positive attitude towards their dietary needs and empower them to advocate for themselves confidently.

7.6 Conclusion

Living gluten-free as a family requires teamwork, patience, and understanding. By educating yourselves about gluten intolerance, creating a gluten-free home environment, advocating for gluten-free accommodations, and providing emotional support to your child, you can help them thrive and lead a happy, healthy life. Remember that you are not alone in your gluten-free journey, and there are resources and support available to help you navigate the challenges and celebrate the joys of raising a gluten-free child.

Chapter 8: Staying Informed and Advocating for Change

Staying informed about gluten-related issues and advocating for change are essential aspects of promoting awareness, understanding, and accessibility for individuals living with gluten intolerance or celiac disease. In this chapter, we'll explore strategies for staying informed, resources for advocacy, and opportunities to effect positive change in the gluten-free community.

8.1 Resources for Staying Informed

Keeping up-to-date on the latest developments in gluten-related research, products, and advocacy efforts is key to staying informed and empowered as a member of the gluten-free community. Here are some resources to consider:

- Celiac disease organizations: Organizations such as the Celiac Disease Foundation, Beyond Celiac, and the Gluten Intolerance Group (GIG) provide valuable information, resources, and support for individuals living with celiac disease and gluten intolerance.
- Medical professionals: Stay connected with healthcare professionals who specialize in celiac disease and gluten-related disorders, such as gastroenterologists, dietitians, and nutritionists, for expert guidance and advice.
- Online communities: Join online forums, social media groups, and discussion boards dedicated to gluten-free living to connect with others, share experiences, and stay informed about the latest news and developments.
- Gluten-free publications: Subscribe to gluten-free magazines, newsletters, and

blogs for articles, recipes, product reviews, and updates on gluten-related topics.

8.2 Advocacy Organizations and Initiatives
Advocacy organizations play a crucial role in raising awareness, promoting research, and advocating for the needs of individuals living with gluten intolerance or celiac disease. Consider getting involved with or supporting organizations that are dedicated to advancing the interests of the gluten-free community, such as:

- Advocacy organizations: Organizations like Beyond Celiac and the Celiac Disease Foundation advocate for policy changes, research funding, and improved access to gluten-free products and accommodations.
- Support groups: Local and national support groups provide a forum for individuals and families affected by celiac disease and gluten intolerance to connect,

share resources, and advocate for change together.
- Legislative initiatives: Stay informed about legislative efforts related to gluten labeling, food safety, and access to gluten-free accommodations in schools, workplaces, and public spaces, and consider supporting or advocating for these initiatives.

8.3 Promoting Awareness and Understanding

Promoting awareness and understanding of gluten intolerance and celiac disease is essential for reducing stigma, dispelling myths, and fostering empathy and support for individuals living with these conditions. Here are some ways to promote awareness:

- Education and outreach: Host educational events, workshops, or presentations in

your community to raise awareness about celiac disease, gluten intolerance, and the gluten-free diet.
- Media campaigns: Use social media, blogs, and other digital platforms to share stories, facts, and resources about living gluten-free and advocate for greater understanding and acceptance.
- Collaboration: Partner with local businesses, schools, healthcare providers, and community organizations to promote gluten-free awareness and support initiatives that benefit the gluten-free community.

8.4 Pushing for Better Labeling and Accessibility
Advocating for better labeling and accessibility of gluten-free products and accommodations is essential for ensuring the safety and well-being of individuals living with gluten intolerance or celiac

disease. Here are some ways to advocate for change:

- Labeling standards: Advocate for clear, accurate, and consistent labeling of gluten-free products to help consumers make informed choices and avoid accidental gluten exposure.
- Accessible options: Push for increased availability of gluten-free options in restaurants, schools, workplaces, healthcare facilities, and public spaces to accommodate individuals with dietary restrictions.
- Policy changes: Advocate for policy changes at the local, state, and federal levels to improve access to gluten-free accommodations, increase funding for celiac disease research, and support initiatives that benefit the gluten-free community.

8.5 Conclusion

Staying informed and advocating for change are powerful ways to support the needs and interests of individuals living with gluten intolerance or celiac disease. By staying connected with resources, supporting advocacy organizations and initiatives, promoting awareness and understanding, and pushing for better labeling and accessibility, you can make a meaningful impact in the gluten-free community and help create a more inclusive and supportive environment for all. Remember that every voice and action counts, and together, we can effect positive change and improve the lives of those affected by gluten-related disorders.

Chapter 9: Overcoming Challenges and Staying Positive

Living gluten-free presents unique challenges, from navigating social situations to managing dietary restrictions in various settings. However, with resilience, support, and a positive mindset, individuals can overcome these challenges and thrive on a gluten-free diet. In this chapter, we'll explore common obstacles faced by those living gluten-free and strategies for maintaining a positive outlook and resilient attitude.

9.1 Dealing with Setbacks and Accidental Gluten Exposure
Despite the best efforts to adhere to a gluten-free diet, setbacks and accidental gluten exposure can occur. Whether it's a mislabeled product, cross-contamination at a restaurant, or a well-meaning but

unaware friend offering you gluten-containing food, it's essential to have strategies in place for coping with these situations. Here are some tips:

- Remain vigilant: Stay educated about hidden sources of gluten and practice reading food labels carefully. Communicate your dietary needs clearly to others and advocate for yourself when necessary.
- Focus on what you can control: While you can't always prevent accidental gluten exposure, you can control how you respond to it. Take proactive steps to mitigate the effects, such as drinking plenty of water, eating simple, gluten-free foods, and practicing self-care to support your well-being.

9.2 Coping with the Psychological Effects of Celiac Disease

Celiac disease can have significant psychological effects on individuals, including feelings of anxiety, frustration, isolation, and even depression. Coping with these emotions is essential for maintaining overall well-being and quality of life. Here are some strategies for managing the psychological effects of celiac disease:

- Seek support: Connect with others who understand what you're going through, whether it's through support groups, online forums, or counseling services. Sharing your experiences with others who can relate can provide validation, empathy, and practical advice.
- Practice self-compassion: Be kind to yourself and acknowledge the challenges you face. Recognize that living with celiac disease requires strength, resilience, and

adaptability, and give yourself credit for your efforts.
- Focus on the positives: While living with celiac disease presents challenges, it also offers opportunities for personal growth, resilience, and self-discovery. Focus on the positives in your life, such as supportive relationships, personal achievements, and the ability to make healthy choices for your well-being.

9.3 Finding Joy and Fulfillment in a Gluten-Free Lifestyle
Living gluten-free doesn't have to be a burden—it can be an opportunity to explore new foods, embrace creativity in the kitchen, and prioritize your health and well-being. Here are some ways to find joy and fulfillment in a gluten-free lifestyle:

- Experiment with new recipes: Get creative in the kitchen and experiment with gluten-free ingredients and recipes. Explore different cuisines, cooking techniques, and flavor combinations to discover delicious, gluten-free meals that you love.

- Focus on whole foods: Emphasize whole, unprocessed foods in your diet, such as fruits, vegetables, lean proteins, and gluten-free grains. Not only are these foods naturally gluten-free, but they also provide essential nutrients and support overall health.

- Celebrate your successes: Take time to celebrate your accomplishments and milestones on your gluten-free journey, whether it's mastering a new recipe, successfully navigating a social event, or simply feeling healthier and more energized.

- Stay connected: Surround yourself with supportive friends, family members, and healthcare professionals who understand and respect your dietary needs. Share your experiences, celebrate your victories, and lean on others for support when needed.

9.4 Conclusion
Living gluten-free presents unique challenges, but with resilience, support, and a positive mindset, individuals can overcome obstacles and thrive on a gluten-free diet. By remaining vigilant, seeking support, practicing self-compassion, and finding joy and fulfillment in a gluten-free lifestyle, you can embrace your dietary needs as a source of strength and empowerment. Remember that you are not alone in your gluten-free journey, and with determination and optimism, you can navigate any challenge and live a vibrant and fulfilling life.

Chapter 10: Looking Ahead: The Future of Gluten-Free Living

As awareness of gluten intolerance and celiac disease continues to grow, the landscape of gluten-free living is evolving rapidly. From advancements in food technology to increased accessibility and support, the future holds promise for individuals living with gluten-related disorders. In this chapter, we'll explore emerging trends, innovations, and opportunities shaping the future of gluten-free living.

10.1 Advancements in Gluten-Free Food Technology

In recent years, there has been a surge in technological advancements aimed at improving the quality, taste, and nutritional profile of gluten-free foods. From innovative ingredient substitutions to novel processing techniques, these advancements are revolutionizing the gluten-free market. Some notable trends include:

- Alternative flours and grains: As demand for gluten-free products continues to rise, manufacturers are exploring alternative flours and grains to diversify their offerings. Look for products made from ancient grains like teff, sorghum, and millet, as well as innovative flour blends that mimic the properties of wheat flour.
- Plant-based proteins: With the growing popularity of plant-based diets, there's an increasing demand for gluten-free plant-based protein sources. Expect to see a rise in plant-based meat alternatives, dairy-free cheeses, and protein-rich snacks made from legumes, nuts, and seeds.
- Clean label ingredients: Consumers are becoming more discerning about the

ingredients in their food, opting for products with clean labels and minimal additives. Manufacturers are responding by reformulating their products to remove artificial flavors, colors, and preservatives, and using natural ingredients to enhance flavor and texture.

10.2 Improved Accessibility and Availability
Accessibility and availability of gluten-free products and accommodations are improving, making it easier for individuals living with gluten-related disorders to navigate everyday life. Some developments to watch for include:

- Expanded product lines: Major food manufacturers and retailers are expanding their gluten-free product lines to meet growing demand. Look for a wider variety of gluten-free options in mainstream

grocery stores, convenience stores, and online retailers.
- Gluten-free labeling standards: Efforts to standardize gluten-free labeling and certification are gaining traction, providing consumers with greater confidence and clarity when choosing gluten-free products. Look for products with certified gluten-free labels or third-party gluten-free certifications.
- Increased awareness and education: Public awareness of celiac disease and gluten intolerance is increasing, thanks to advocacy efforts, media coverage, and educational campaigns. As a result, more people are recognizing the importance of gluten-free accommodations and supporting initiatives to improve accessibility and inclusivity.

10.3 Supportive Communities and Resources

Supportive communities and resources play a crucial role in helping individuals living with gluten-related disorders navigate their dietary needs and find support and encouragement. Some emerging trends in this area include:

- Online communities and social media: Social media platforms and online forums provide a forum for individuals to connect, share experiences, and offer support to others living with gluten-related disorders. Look for Facebook groups, Instagram accounts, and dedicated websites and blogs focused on gluten-free living.
- Telehealth and virtual support: Telehealth services and virtual support groups are becoming increasingly popular, providing convenient access to healthcare professionals, dietitians, and support networks from the comfort of home. Look for telehealth platforms and online support

groups tailored to individuals living with celiac disease and gluten intolerance.

10.4 The future of gluten-free living is bright, with advancements in food technology, improved accessibility and availability, and supportive communities and resources empowering individuals living with gluten-related disorders to thrive. By staying informed, embracing innovation, and advocating for change, we can create a more inclusive and supportive environment for all. As we look ahead, let's continue to work together to ensure that everyone has the opportunity to enjoy a vibrant and fulfilling life, free from the constraints of gluten intolerance and celiac disease.

Conclusion: Embracing Your Gluten-Free Journey

Living gluten-free isn't just about dietary restrictions—it's a journey of self-discovery, resilience, and empowerment. In this chapter, we'll explore the importance of embracing your gluten-free journey, celebrating your successes, and finding joy and fulfillment in the process.

Embracing self-discovery and living with gluten intolerance or celiac disease often requires a period of adjustment and self-discovery as you navigate your dietary needs and learn to advocate for yourself. Embrace this journey of self-discovery as an opportunity to explore new foods, cooking techniques, and lifestyle habits that support your health and well-being. Take the time to listen to your body, tune into your unique nutritional needs, and discover what works best for you.

<u>Cultivating Resilience and Adaptability</u>
Living gluten-free requires resilience and adaptability in the face of challenges and setbacks. Embrace the opportunity to cultivate these qualities as you navigate the ups and downs of your gluten-free journey. Remember that setbacks are a natural part of the process and an opportunity for growth and learning. Approach challenges with a positive mindset, knowing that you have the strength and resilience to overcome them.

<u>Celebrating Your Successes</u>
Take time to celebrate your successes, big and small, on your gluten-free journey. Whether it's mastering a new gluten-free recipe, successfully navigating a social event, or simply feeling healthier and more

energized, each achievement deserves recognition and celebration. Celebrate your progress, acknowledge your efforts, and take pride in how far you've come on your gluten-free journey.

Finding Joy and Fulfillment
Living gluten-free doesn't have to be a burden—it can be a source of joy, fulfillment, and empowerment. Embrace the opportunity to explore new foods, flavors, and cuisines that nourish your body and delight your taste buds. Focus on the positive aspects of your gluten-free lifestyle, such as improved health, increased energy, and a greater appreciation for wholesome, nourishing foods.

Connecting with Others
Building a supportive community of friends, family members, healthcare professionals,

and fellow gluten-free individuals can make a world of difference on your gluten-free journey. Embrace the opportunity to connect with others who understand what you're going through, share experiences, and offer support and encouragement. Whether it's joining a local support group, attending gluten-free events, or connecting with others online, finding your tribe can provide a sense of belonging and camaraderie.

11.6 Conclusion
Embracing your gluten-free journey is about more than just managing dietary restrictions—it's about embracing a lifestyle of self-discovery, resilience, and empowerment. By cultivating resilience, celebrating your successes, finding joy and fulfillment, and connecting with others, you can navigate your gluten-free journey with confidence and grace. Remember that

every challenge you overcome and every success you achieve is a testament to your strength and resilience. Embrace your gluten-free journey as an opportunity for growth, transformation, and self-discovery, and let it enrich your life in ways you never imagined possible.